583797

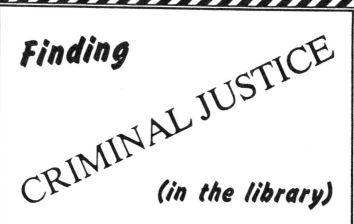

Finding CRIMINAL JUSTICE (in the library)

A Student Manual of Information Retrieval
and Utilization Skills

Dennis C. Tucker

Frank Schmalleger

 Wyndham Hall Press

FINDING CRIMINAL JUSTICE (IN THE LIBRARY)

A Student Manual of Information Retrieval
and Utilization Skills

by

Dennis C. Tucker & Frank Schmalleger

Dennis C. Tucker, Series Editor

(Titles Projected in the Series)

FINDING RELIGION (in the library)
FINDING PSYCHOLOGY (in the library)
FINDING POLITICAL SCIENCE (in the library)
FINDING SOCIOLOGY (in the library)
FINDING CRIMINAL JUSTICE (in the library)
FINDING ECONOMICS (in the library)
FINDING EDUCATION (in the library)
FINDING ENGLISH LITERATURE (in the library)
FINDING BUSINESS (in the library)
FINDING NURSING (in the library)
FINDING PHILOSOPHY (in the library)

ISBN 1-55605-183-2 paperback
ISBN 1-55605-184-0 hardback

TABLE OF CONTENTS

INTRODUCTION

A wise person once said, "Give a man a fish and you feed him for a day; teach him to fish and you feed him for a lifetime."

Educators have often been told that we teach people, not subjects. Yet, if we teach a person a subject, we still have not fulfilled our mission. We must teach him or her how to learn that subject without assistance from us. He or she needs to progress beyond the limit of our knowledge. A good foundation in research skills is, therefore, an essential part of a good education and one that will last a lifetime.

Our years of experience both in teaching and in library work have shown us that we educators have often failed in teaching research skills. It is the purpose of this book, part of the **Library Research** series, to provide instruction in the basic skills necessary for doing research in the area of Criminal Justice. We are going to look at libraries and how they can be used to the best advantage. We will attempt to offer some basic resources and techniques which can be used by the student of Criminal Justice while in school and later by the graduate--the professional, the police officer, the judicial administrator, the correctional officer, etc.--who no longer has access to a teacher or faculty member for direction but must gather information independently.

We will discuss, explain, and demonstrate five major components essential to the responsible development of information retrieval and utilization skills in the field of Criminal Justice.

FIRST, we will look at the overall **layout of the library** itself (at whatever college or university). We will discuss the organization of the holdings and their various categories and functions. We will list and explain the various staff positions typical in a college or university library, and we will make some references to general policies of utilization most commonly found in such libraries.

SECOND, we will examine the old standby, **the card catalog**, and its smallest unit, the catalog card. Each card contains a wealth of information that many non-librarians don't even know exists and can serve as a springboard to a vast pool of other resources.

THIRD, we will consider the reference collection and briefly discuss what distinguishes a reference book from a non-reference book. At the same time, we will outline some basic criteria for evaluating a reference work, and look at some of the **major reference sources** in the subject area of Criminal Justice.

FOURTH, the professional who wishes to keep current in his field must know how to use **the periodical literature** to locate the latest research. We will look at periodicals and their indexes--both the traditional manual indexes and their newer counterparts, automated indexes.

FINALLY, we will briefly discuss and illustrate a very effective method of **research documentation** and discuss ways of **developing a research paper** from the choice of the initial topic to its completion.

We will take a look at the most valuable library resource of all--the library staff, and especially, the reference librarian. This information professional is a trained researcher with skills that will allow him to locate information in any field, be it theology, philosophy, medicine, law, or engineering. Nowadays, the well prepared reference librarian is not only a researcher, but an expert in logic (Boolean, to be precise), information management, and in computer systems.

When we began graduate school we experienced an over-whelming feeling of awe every time we entered the library--so much knowledge contained therein and we would only be able to begin to scratch the surface. As time went by, we came to the conclusion that probably one percent of that volume was fresh knowledge and the rest repetition. As we developed our research skills, our final conclusion was that, though we could never learn it all, with the proper tools we could find any single piece or pieces of information that we wanted; the rest didn't interest us anyway. In short, our research ability allowed us to separate the wheat from the chaff. It is the hope of authors and publisher that the titles in this series will help the beginning researcher develop the same skills.

CHAPTER ONE

THE LIBRARY--IT'S OUT THERE SOMEWHERE

Just as a person wishing to drive must first find a car, so one seeking an education must begin by finding the seat of learning--the library. One of the first things the conscientious student will want to do soon after registering is to find the campus library. Often the building will be easy to spot just because of its size and architectural style, but sometimes it won't be. Ask around. Usually there is at least one student on campus who has visited the library sometime during his college career and he or she will be glad to help you find it.

Once you have located the library, we suggest a visit--actually going there when you don't have to!--just to have a look around. Just browse to get a general idea of the layout. Locate the various stack areas and the different types of collections that are contained within the building. Find the bathrooms and water fountains and the quiet areas for study. Perhaps now is a good time to locate a favorite hideaway that will later become your special secret place for studying.

Some libraries will have printed brochures which give information on the library, telling about its various collections, special display areas, where various parts of the collection are located, etc. If you don't see such a brochure, ask the library personnel if one is available.

Other libraries are even more elaborate in orienting new users to the library. An increasing number of libraries are using audio or video cassettes for orientation. It is sometimes possible to check out a videotape for home use. Other times, libraries may have a special viewing area where you can go to watch the tape which is, in essence, a guided tour of the building.

Some libraries have audio tapes which you can borrow along with a cassette player for in-house use. These tapes contain a self-guided tour of the library. You play the tape and follow its directions for a walking tour of the building.

And some libraries have personnel who will give you a guided tour of the building. Depending upon the policy of the library, a tour may be available on demand or at specified times, in which case you can sign up to come back later and join a group. Most colleges and universities have some type of library tour (often called "bibliographic instruction tour" or "freshmen orientation tour") for freshmen and new students.

The introductory visit to the library is a good time to acquaint yourself with its particular policies and procedures. What types of materials can be checked out? For how long? How do you get a library card? What types of materials must be used in-house? What are the library hours? Is there an after-hours study area? What is the availability of special collections, inter-library loan, computer databases? The more you know about the building and its layout, the more comfortable you will feel using its services and dealing with its personnel.

A good library contains more than just books. It will have a variety of educational materials, aids, and services with a staff of professionally trained individuals who are happy to assist the inquiring student seeking to utilize its resources.

There is a logic to the arrangement of the materials and an organization of the various functions of the staff. The serious student will acquaint himself with the library, its methods, concepts and procedures.

At this point, it will be helpful to point out the fundamental structure of the holdings and the staff positions of the typical college library.

Not everyone who works in a doctor's office is a doctor. Neither is everyone who works in a library a librarian.

Just as you would not expect the doctor's cashier to perform surgery, you should not expect a library page to have the answer to an involved reference question.

Within the library are clerks, staff assistants, secretaries, pages, student workers, and librarians. The librarian is a professional with a minimum of an accredited Master's Degree in Library Science. Most institutions of higher education have the same requirements for a librarian as for a member of the teaching faculty. A second Master's Degree is often required for tenure.

Libraries are organized in many different ways, depending on their size and the needs of the patrons or institution they serve. But, generally speaking, libraries are organized into two broad areas, **TECHNICAL SERVICES** and **PUBLIC SERVICES.**

TECHNICAL SERVICES

Technical services staff can be thought of as those who work behind the scenes. They are the ones responsible for ordering the materials (though not necessarily deciding **which** materials to order) and handling them from the time they arrive at the delivery dock until they are on the shelf. Technical services is divided into several major areas:

Acquisitions. Those in the acquisitions department actually place the orders for the materials with the various publishers and suppliers. When the materials arrive, it is their responsibility to receive them, make sure that the order has arrived as requested, pass on the invoices for payment and the materials for processing.

Cataloging. The cataloging department is responsible for the organization of the collection. It is their duty to see that materials on the same subject are grouped together on the shelf to make it easier for the patron to find them. Therefore, they classify the materials and assign call numbers according to whichever classification system the library uses (usually the Dewey Decimal System or the Library of Congress System).

The cataloging department is responsible for preparing entries for each book for the card catalog (or the automated catalog, if there is one) and filing the cards in the drawers. They are also responsible for the process in reverse--removing entries from the catalog for materials that have been lost or discarded.

Processing. Some libraries have a processing department which is responsible for the physical preparation of the material. They do such tasks as applying spine labels and barcodes (if used), inserting book pockets, and placing plastic covers on the books.

Mending and binding. This department, sometimes combined with and sometimes separate from processing, is responsible for the physical well-being of the materials. Worn and torn materials are mended and repaired. Larger libraries may have their own in-house bindery. Most libraries send materials needing extensive repair to an outside bindery. It is the responsibility of this department to get them there and back.

Serials. Serials are materials that come at repeated intervals--such as yearbooks or magazines. This department is responsible for receiving the materials when they arrive, checking them in and getting them to the shelf. It is also their responsibility to notice materials which fail to arrive and contact the supplier. In larger libraries **Periodicals** (magazines) may be a separate department from or a subdivision of the serials department.

PUBLIC SERVICES

The people in the **public services** are the ones you will usually see in your visits to the library. Their primary function is to assist you, the patron.

One of the major subdivisions of the Public Services department is the **circulation department.** This department is primarily responsible for checking out materials to the borrower and getting them back. When materials are returned, it is their job to get them back to the proper shelf. If the library uses a fine system, they must collect the fines for overdue materials. If materials are not returned, it is the responsibility of the circulation department to contact the recalcitrant borrower and, occasionally, turn over the case to a collection agency.

The reserve book department may be contained within or be separate from the circulation department. A professor may make a reading assignment for an entire class (or several classes) in the same book. If there is only one copy of the book in the library and someone checks it out, no one else gets a chance to read the assignment. To avoid this, the professor may choose to place the book on reserve. Reserve simply means that the book is placed on limited circulation. Instead of being checked out for the usual two, three or four weeks at a time (whatever the policy of the library is), the book may now be checked out only for overnight use or for two hours' use within the library. (Again, this time period varies according to the policy of each library and the wishes of the professor.) Its purpose is to make a limited number of materials available to the greatest number of users within the shortest period of time.

The Reference Department is probably the department (other than circulation) that the student will deal with the most. As hard as it may be to believe, libraries actually pay someone for sitting at a desk and answering questions. This person is available and waiting to be asked.

It is a misconception that this is someone who was stuck out there at the desk because he didn't know how to do anything else, so the library gave him or her the only job that was available. In fact, quite the contrary is true. The reference librarian is perhaps the most highly trained individual in the library. It is he or she who knows the collection and the tools for accessing it. The reference librarian with a second Master's may also be a scholar in his or her own particular academic discipline. He or she can be the researcher's single most valuable asset.

While it is impossible for an individual reference librarian to be an expert in every single subject area in which someone may require assistance, he is trained in the technique of locating information. Though the sources are not the same for all disciplines, the technique is. The reference librarian is trained in the basic sources for all disciplines or at least knows which tools to use to find them. Larger libraries have a staff of reference librarians, each with his own subject specialties; if one can't help, possibly another one can.

Before approaching the reference librarian, there is a basic supposition which must be understood: This individual is there to help you do your work, not to do it for you. Exhaust your own resources before asking for assistance, so that you may say, "I've looked in the card catalog for books on Criminal Justice, but I couldn't find any. Am I looking under the right subject heading?"

Be as specific as possible in your request. Don't say, "Where are your Criminal Justice books?" Say, "I'm trying to locate the original text of Sutherland's **Criminology**. Can you tell me where I might look?"

Expect the reference librarian to answer your question with a question. He is trained to elicit as much information from you as possible so that he may be as specific as possible in finding the answer you want. He is not trying to pry, only to be specific. If the information you are researching is confidential, say so. Most librarians couldn't care less what you are researching, but they do need as much information as you can give them so they can be sure of finding the right answer for you.

After the librarian has helped you, if the answer is not what you need, feel free to say, "Thank you, but that's not quite what I'm looking for. Is there another source we could check?" The reference librarian wants to find the answer, but often doesn't know if he's succeeded unless you tell him.

Be courteous in your use of the reference librarian's time. The reference desk, particularly in an academic library, can be busier than New Orleans at Mardi Gras. It is not unusual in some libraries to see four or five people in line and two phones ringing at the same time. Try to keep your query as brief and as simple as possible. If your question requires an in-depth answer which is going to take some time, schedule your time at the reference desk when it is less busy. Some reference desks will even make an appointment for you to have a lengthy session with the person who is most skilled in your subject area.

Begin your work on time. A favorite complaint of teachers is heard even more often by reference librarians: "I have this termpaper due tomorrow and I need five sources." Locating information takes time. After it's found, it most likely will not be in the form you need for your paper. It's going to take some time for you to pull it together and reorganize it. Remember that the responsibility of the reference librarian ends with locating the information; he should not be expected to explain something which you are supposed to understand on your own nor to write your termpaper for you.

It is fair to expect the reference librarian to teach you how to use the card catalog or to show you where the books are found. It is not fair to ask the librarian to look up every book or to retrieve it for you. If you don't understand something about the library, ask, but ask with the goal of learning to do it for yourself.

Many libraries offer telephone reference service. These libraries will take a phone call and give you a specific piece of information over the phone. By all means, use the service, but do not abuse it.

Keep your query to a simple fact or two. The telephone reference staff will be glad to tell you the current population of New York City or whether or not the library has a certain book (and in some cases whether it's checked out or not), but don't expect them to have time to read you a four-page essay over the phone.

If it sounds like the library is busy, keep your phone query brief or ask if there is a more convenient time for you to call back. Traffic at the reference desk seems to go in spurts: The librarian may sit for ten or fifteen minutes with no questions and suddenly six people approach at the same time--all of them with lengthy requests. Most libraries give priority to the patron who has put forth the effort to go in person over the one making a convenient phone call from home. For questions that are a little lengthy, some libraries will be glad to take your phone number and call you back.

If the library doesn't own the book you need or seems to have nothing on your topic, ask the reference librarian if they have **Inter-Library Loan service.** This service provides access to books from other libraries where you would not normally be allowed borrowing privileges. Again, be as specific as possible with your request. Some libraries will only handle a request for a specific book, while others are prepared to fill a subject request.

Always allow two to three weeks for an Inter-Library Loan request. Remember that your library is at the mercy of the lending library, so don't get upset with your library if the book is slow in coming. Ask what the usual response time is; then, if you haven't heard by that time, inquire again. If the lending period is short, that has been deter-mined by the lending library, not by your library. If renewals are not allowed, that is the policy of the lender, not of your library.

Another department under the umbrella of **Public Services** may be the **Database Search** department. It may be called

Online Searching, Information Retrieval or a myriad of other names. Many of the indexes which were previously available only in paper form, plus many new ones, are now available in electronic format. Depending on the complexity of your search and the type of information you need, this may be the quickest and best way to locate the information. If you think you might need the service, ask if it's available.

Larger libraries often have a department devoted specifically to **bibliographic instruction,** teaching about books and libraries--your library in particular. It is this department which conducts the orientation tours for new students and provides materials to professors for use in teaching about the library in the classroom. If you want to learn how to use the library to your best advantage, someone from this department can work with you.

Another major department is **periodicals.** We discussed previously the portion of the periodicals department which is responsible for receiving the materials and getting them to the shelves. This is the portion which handles the materials once they are on the shelf and available to the user.

Periodicals are generally divided into two sections: current periodicals and older issues. In most libraries, the current issues are in an area by themselves. The majority of libraries simply place the materials on the shelf in alphabetical order by the title of the magazine or journal. Some libraries, however, classify them and assign a call number so that all journals on the same subject are shelved near each other. In this case, you will need to use a catalog to find the call number so you can locate the journal.

The type of catalog used for journals varies from library to library. Some libraries will simply keep a printed list or a computer printout listing the journals that are held. Often, additional information is given, such as the volume numbers and dates of each title owned by the library. Other libraries use a "visible file," which is a kind of chart listing the titles in alphabetical sequence. Each title is held in a strip of plastic and the chart may be updated with relative ease as titles are added or dropped. Still other libraries list their journals in the card catalog, so the user must go there to find out if the library owns a particular title and its call number if materials are classified.

Older materials are often moved to a separate area of the library. (The definition of older varies widely from one library to another, but very generally, it means anything prior to the current year.) Some libraries bind their magazines so the issues stay together in order and are easier to shelve and locate. To many new users, the shelves look like they are full of books, but a glance inside the covers will show you that they are just the magazines you are familiar with, sewn together at the spine, and a hard book-like cover added to them.

Other libraries simply box the materials so that the issues of a given volume are shelved together in the same box. And some libraries discard their paper copies of journals altogether and keep back issues only on microfilm or microfiche. Within a given library, it is not unusual to find materials treated all four ways: some bound, some boxed, some on microfilm, and some on microfiche.

Depending on the library, the section for bound journals may be a special section housing only journals, as is usually the case. Some libraries, however, classify and catalog the older issues just as they would a book. So, a medical journal will be found shelved in the regular stacks right next to the medical books.

Somewhere near the periodicals you will usually find the **periodicals indexes.** If you are trying to find an article on C. S. Lewis, for example, you could just go to a journal where you think the article might have appeared and flip through the issues until you found it, but such a procedure would probably require a great deal of time and effort unless you were sure of the exact magazine and knew the issue it appeared in. A much easier way is to locate a periodicals index and look under "Lewis, C. S." or whatever subject you need to locate. There, you will find the title of the journal the article appeared in, its author, the issue it appeared in, and the pages on which it appeared. We will discuss periodicals indexes in greater depth in chapter four.

Many libraries, especially larger ones, have a collection of **government documents.** Despite the awe-inspiring title, these are nothing more than a collection of items which are published by federal, state, and local government bodies. Each year government organizations publish many thousands of documents. Some libraries are defined as "depository libraries," which means they automatically receive all or a selected portion of these items. Because there are so many items, it could be a time-consuming and overwhelming task to classify all of them and add them to the regular collection. So, some libraries simply designate a special area for them and use the classification scheme which has been established by the government. While quite different from the Dewey or Library of Congress system, it is no more difficult, and you should learn to use it early if you think you will need government publications in your research--and chances are most of us will.

In addition to the above departments which are found in most every library, your library may have other special departments. Sometimes these are classed under the title of **Special Collections** and may include rare books; the college archives; denominational archives, if the institution is affiliated with a particular religious body; the collected works of a particular author; a genealogy collection; or a local history collection. There are many types of special collections and some may be unique to an institution. Ask which ones your library has.

Get to know your library and its staff early in your educational career. Eventually you will find that knowing how to locate information in the library is even more important than what you'll learn in the classroom. Your classroom

instruction will last four or five years before being outdated
or forgotten. Using the library is a skill that will last a
lifetime. Your library and its staff are there to serve you.
Use them. And don't forget to say, "Thanks."

CHAPTER TWO

THE CARD CATALOG

Just as a telescope is one of the keys to the universe, so is the card catalog one of the keys to the library. Learn to use it.

The card catalog provides three points of access to the library collection: It lists books by their author, their title, and their subject matter. Some libraries use a "dictionary" catalog in which all three types of cards are filed in a single alphabet. Other libraries use a divided catalog with each type of card filed in a separate alphabet in a separate cabinet or set of cabinets. In other libraries, author and title cards are filed together and subject cards are filed in a separate alphabet. It is vital for you to know which type of system a library uses before beginning your research.

It is also important to know which type of filing system your library uses. Most libraries use word-by-word filing and follow a rule we call the "nothing before something" rule. In a word-by-word system, for example, the subject "New York" would file before "Newark" or "Newsweek" because "nothing"--the blank space between the two words--files before "something"--the letter "a" or the letter's." This rule is becoming increasingly important to understand with the advent of automation because a computer will alphabetize "nothing" before "something".

Another important filing rule is the "by before about" rule. All the books **by** an author are filed in the catalog before books **about** him. Likewise, a book written by "Brown, Zelda" would file before a book entitled **The Brown Boat.**

There is also a hierarchy of filing rules as to which comes first of commas, periods, colons, semi-colons, and hyphens.

Generally, a library user need not be concerned with such intricate detail other than to know that if you don't find the book listed where you think it should be, try another likely spot. If you have trouble locating a book, inquire which system your library uses or ask the reference librarian for help.

The individual unit of the catalog is the catalog card. Being able to read and understand the information contained on a card will unleash great research power.

A card is divided into paragraphs. Each paragraph is indented and contains specific information. Author, title, and subject cards are virtually alike, but different information is printed at the top of the card.

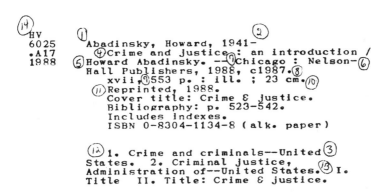

Figure 1.

AUTHOR. Figure 1 is a sample of a catalog card for Howard Abadinsky's **Crime and Justice.** The first paragraph of a catalog card always begins with the last name of the **author**(1), if there is an author. When there is no author, the title of the work appears first. This card is what we call an author card. Note that the birth and death dates of the author are sometimes given.(2) This helps the researcher distinguish between people of the same name. (Try looking in the card catalog of a large library for John Kennedy.) The author card is usually called the "main entry" and may sometimes contain more information than a title or subject card. If the work has no author, the title card is considered the main entry.

SUBJECT. If this were a subject card, the subject "Crime and criminals--United States" or "Criminal justice, Administration of--United States"(3) would be typed at the very top of the card above the author paragraph in all capital letters. Some catalogs still contain older cards on which the subjects were typed at the top using red ink, but current practice is to use all-caps. Either red ink or all-caps indicates that this is the subject, not the title, of the book. A **subject** may be a topic per se, or it may be the name of a person, place or thing.

TITLE. Below the author's name, and indented, is the **title** of the book.(4) If this were a title card, the title would be repeated at the top of the card above the author's name. Note that the title is neither typed in red nor in all capital letters and that usually only the first word and proper nouns are capitalized. (This style of non-capitalization is followed simply to increase the cataloger's typing speed by not having to press the "shift" key repeatedly.)

STATEMENT OF RESPONSIBILITY. Immediately following the title and in the same paragraph is what is called the **statement of responsibility** which is usually a repetition of the author's name and may include co-authors, editors, translators(5) or illustrators. Next, and in the same paragraph, is the **imprint.** The imprint is information specific to this edition of the book. If this is at least the second edition of a book, it will list here which edition this is. The **imprint** contains the publisher's name(6) and location(7), and the copyright date of the book.(8) The researcher can use information from the imprint to determine the nationality of a publication. A book published in Ireland may not give a proper perspective of some American event, but it may be the best source for something that occurred in Ireland. A glance at the publisher's name may tell the researcher something about the quality of this book. And the copyright date will show how current the information is.

COLLATION. The paragraph after the imprint is the **collation.** If the paragraph begins with a lower case Roman numeral, that tells how many pages of introductory material are contained in the work. An Arabic numeral(9) shows the number of pages in the body of the work. The statement "il.," "ill." or "illus." indicates that the book contains illustrations. If you must have a picture of the person or subject you are researching and this statement is absent, obviously you should look for another source. Often the statement is so specific as to indicate that the book contains maps, charts, graphs or other specific types of illustrative material. And finally, many cards give the height of the book in centimeters.(10) Generally of interest to librarians for shelving purposes, this statement may give you an overall idea of the size of the book you are dealing with. You won't want to plan on walking home or riding the bus with a stack of books that are 96 centimeters tall.

NOTES. Following the collation is the **notes** paragraph.(11) If the book has an index or a bibliography, it is listed here. Many cards list the page number on which this information is given. With this information, a researcher can quickly locate a book which he might have overlooked as being of no value in itself for his project, but the bibliography of which may prove invaluable in locating further sources (or "primary" or original sources) on the subject. Some cards may give additional notes about the work such as a brief summary of the book or some type of information particular to this edition or even this copy such as "autographed by the author." A special note, for instance may show that the book was originally published under another title.

TRACINGS. The last paragraph on the card is called the **tracings.**(12) Those items which appear following Arabic numerals are subject headings under which this book is listed in the card catalog.(3) They are extremely helpful to the researcher wishing to locate similar books or other books on the same topic. Simply make note of what seems to be a promising subject heading and look in the catalog under that heading. Items which appear after Roman numerals(13) are called "added entries" and refer to such things as co-authors, illustrators, alternate titles or the series of which the book forms a part, if any. The researcher wishing to find similar books might want to look elsewhere in the catalog under the name of the co-author or the series.

CALL NUMBER. Finally, in the upper left hand corner of the card is the "call number"(14) which tells where the book is located on the shelf. In most American libraries this number will belong either to the "Dewey Decimal" system or the "Library of Congress" system.

A Dewey number will have a first line which consists of numerals only with exactly three digits to the left of the decimal point. The second line is a **Cutter number,** which is a mixture of letters and numbers representing the author's last name and the title of the work. Generally speaking, a Cutter number will begin with a capital letter (the first letter of the author's last name) followed by two or three digits, followed by a lower case letter which is the first letter of the first significant word of the title.

A typical Dewey number would appear like this:

Subject number	618.2
Cutter number	M484r

An LC number will consist of a subject number, comprised of both letters and numerals and a Cutter number. An LC number always begins with a letter or two. The Cutter number is preceded by a decimal point. (An LC number may contain several decimal points, while a Dewey number may contain only one.) A typical LC number would appear thus:

> Subject number   PS 613
> Cutter number   .W47

In both systems the Cutter number is treated as a decimal, so that on the shelf a book with the LC number "PS613.W47" would come before "PS613.W5". A book with the Dewey number "618.2 M484r" would come before "618.2 M53j".

For a basic introduction to the library and classification systems, the student is well advised to take a careful look at Jean Key Gates' **Guide to the Use of Libraries and Information Sources,** 6th edition. (New York: McGraw-Hill, 1988.) and the **Dewey Decimal Classification and Relative Index.**

THE LIBRARY OF CONGRESS CLASSIFICATION SYSTEM

In 1897 the task of recataloging and reclassifying the Library of Congress was begun. The Library of Congress Classification System, which was developed in that process, combines letters of the alphabet and Arabic numerals; it provides for the most minute groupings of subjects through the combination of letters and numerals; it is designed for libraries with very large collections. The letters I, O, W, X, and Y are not used but are left for further expansion.

A brief outline of the Library of Congress Classification System follows:

A   General Works - Polygraphy

B   Philosophy - Religion

C   History - Auxiliary sciences

D   History and Topography (except America)

E-F   America

G   Geography - Anthropology

H   Social Sciences

J   Political Science

K   Law

L   Education

M   Music

N   Fine Arts

P   Language and Literature

Q   Science

R   Medicine

S   Agriculture - Plant and Animal Industry

T   Technology

U   Military Science

V   Naval Science

Z   Bibliography and Library Science

Because Criminal Justice is a very broad and diverse subject area, materials related to the topic are located in a wide variety of call numbers. Generally speaking, the subject of Criminal Justice falls within the area of the social sciences, which uses the "H" schedule of LC classification. The breakdown of the "H" schedule is as follows:

H   Social sciences (general)

HA   Statistics

HB   Economic theory

HC   Economic history and conditions

HD   Economic history and conditions

HE   Transportation and communications

HF   Commerce

HG   Finance

HJ   Public finance

HM   Sociology

HN   Social History and conditions. Social problems. Social Reform.

HQ   The family. Marriage. Woman.

HS   Societies: Secret, benevolent, etc.

HT   Communities. Classes. Races.

HU   Crime and criminals. Social pathology.

HV   Social pathology. Social and public welfare. Criminology.

HX   Socialism. Communism. Anarchism.

The majority of materials on criminal justice will be located in the "HU" or "HV" area. Since there is much crossover into the legal world, many appropriate materials may also be found in the "K" schedule.

There are many other sub-categories within these divisions. These will give the student some exposure to the sophistication and detailed specialization that library science has brought to the cataloging of books in modern times.

THE DEWEY DECIMAL CLASSIFICATION SYSTEM

In the Dewey Decimal Classification System, Arabic numerals are used to signify the various classes of subjects.

Melvil Dewey divided all knowledge, as represented by books and other materials, into nine classes which he numbered 100 to 900. Materials too general to belong in a specific group, such as encyclopedias, dictionaries, newspapers, handbooks, and the like, he placed in a tenth class, which precedes the others as the 000 class. Every student should know these ten categories. They are part of the basic knowledge of research, and the student will use this information at every library using the Dewey Decimal Classification System. These ten major categories are:

000   General Works

100   Philosophy

200   Religion

300   Social Sciences

400   Language

500   Pure Science

600   Technology, Applied Science

700   The Arts

800   Literature

900   History, Biography

The system progresses from the preceding ten general classifications to more and more precise subclassifications, based on a decade arrangement. Each of the above ten categories is again divided into ten subcategories, thus providing 100 slots into which books may be classified. Each of these 100 slots is again divided into ten further classification areas.

Usually, this three-digit hundred category is followed by a decimal point, after which the subdividing continues. As you can see from the above chart, the major category for Criminal Justice is the 300s, as it is one of the social sciences. Materials that relate to legal matters are classified in the 340s, and those dealing with social pathology and services, including criminology and penal and related institutions, are classed in the 360s.

Both systems are simply ways of classifying information so that books on a given topic are placed near each other on the shelf. This, in turn, makes it easier for the user to locate other books on the chosen subject. While smaller libraries tend to use Dewey and larger libraries LC, there is no rule, and it actually makes little difference to the user.

Some libraries handle biography and autobiography a little differently from other types of nonfiction. Instead of being assigned a call number, biographies may simply be marked with a "B" and shelved in a separate section. Other libraries use "921" or simply a "92" (from the Dewey Decimal system) to indicate biography. Usually they are filed by last name of the **subject** (not the author), so, all biographies about Lincoln would appear together on the shelf. If biographies aren't where it seems they should be, ask where they are shelved.

Some libraries shelve fiction in a separate section. Instead of a call number, an "F" or "Fic" appears in the upper left hand corner of the card and the books are then filed by author's last name in the fiction section. Other libraries don't bother to indicate "F" or "Fic" and the corner of the card appears blank, indicating simply that books are filed in the fiction section by author's last name. In some libraries, some works of fiction may be classified as literature and shelved with the regular collection under the appropriate call number for literature.

Where do you begin if you don't know what the proper subject heading is for a topic? How do you know whether to look under "Railroad trains," "Trains," "Trains, Railroad," "Passenger trains," "Passenger service--rail," "Trains, Passenger," or "Railroads, Passenger"? If library catalogers filed a card under whatever subject heading appealled to them at the moment, it would be difficult to locate all the books in the library on a given subject, particularly over the years as there were staff changes in the cataloging department. Therefore, catalogers use a guide entitled **Library of Congress Subject Headings** for the specific purpose of providing standardization. If you're not sure what the proper subject heading is, look in **LC**--a large red book, usually in two volumes--under what you feel is the most likely. **LC** provides ample cross references to the correct heading. (Proper headings are printed in **Boldface** print.) Many libraries keep a copy near the card catalog or at the reference desk. If you don't see a copy of **LC**, ask at the reference desk.

Many libraries are now automating their catalogs. This process allows greater flexibility in manipulating information and a larger number of access points for the user. Some systems even contain circulation information so the user knows immediately if the desired book is on the shelf or checked out. Often the information on the computer screen will look similar to that on a catalog card.

Whichever system your library uses, introduce yourself early and become familiar with it. A couple of hours "playing" in the library when you don't need to will be an invaluable timesaver when that termpaper is due tomorrow.

CHAPTER THREE

The Reference Collection -- Tomes of Information

Often due to a lack of basic knowledge of library usage, a student will assume the library deficient in materials when, in reality, there is a mountain of literature that is inaccessible to the unskilled user. Nowhere in the library is there to be found such a concentration of research materials as in the **Reference Department.** Here, among other resources, are to be found dictionaries (there is really more than one kind!), encyclopedias (they are not all the same!), government documents (it is actually possible to read and understand them), and a full range of indices (the plural form of "index"). We will discuss these groupings below, but first, let's take a closer look at reference books in general.

EVALUATING A REFERENCE BOOK

What is a reference book? What distinguishes it from a non-reference book?

A primary distinction is revealed by the term itself: a reference book is not intended to be read from cover to cover like a novel or a biography, but is **referred to** in order to locate specific factual information. The information is usually, but not always, brief in nature.

Having determined what a reference book is, how does one determine what a **good** reference book is? There are a number of criteria which may be applied.

First of all, read the introductory material. Usually there is a section (or sections) at the beginning of the work which tells it purpose, its scope, and briefly outlines it contents.

Knowing the authors' purpose, we can then apply other criteria to decide whether or not they fulfill that purpose.

Scope. The scope of a book is its span of coverage. In order to locate information efficiently we must determine whether a particular book deals adequately with the topic we are investigating. A book entitled **America in the Twenties** would probably be limited to a discussion of things happening in America during the 1920s and would not be our primary text for research on European current events during World War II. Its scope includes neither the topic we are researching (Europe) nor the time period (World War II).

Bias. Bias is not always a negative term. We all have bias; some of us just won't admit it. However, when an author's point of view is limited by the purposeful exclusion of any evidence which disagrees with his opinion, we can say that he is biased. The distinction between a biased work and an unbiased one is sometimes thin, but essentially, if an author presents his viewpoint as **his viewpoint**, we can say the work is unbiased. If he presents his viewpoint as the absolute truth, willfully excluding or ignoring abundant evidence to the contrary, we can say the work is biased. In researching the history of a particular church denomination, for example, a text written by a member of that denomination may be the best source, for a member can have a feeling and an appreciation for the denomination that an outsider cannot. If, however, the author's zeal for promoting the denomination distorts the facts, a text written by an outside party may be the best source.

Point of view. Every book has a point of view. In order to determine whether a book suits our research purpose, we must determine what that point of view is. The author might be looking at his subject from either the inside or the outside--a member of a group or an outsider writing its history. His purpose might be to convert or simply to lay down the facts. An author's timeframe is also a point of view. A book like the above-mentioned **America**

in the Twenties could either be a look at current events or a historical perspective of the decade, depending upon when it was written and the point of view of the author. Either point of view is valid, but either one may not suit our purpose. In choosing a reference book, we must make sure that the author's point of view is appropriate to the subject and to our needs.

Copyright. The copyright date of a work can often tell us immediately if it is the source we need. If the piece of information we need is the number of persons in prison in the United States at year-end 1990, a book with a 1967 copyright date will give us the wrong information. Though perfectly correct when the book was published, time has made the information false if we need a current figure. On the other hand, if we are researching changes in incarceration rates over the last few decades, the 1967 figure may be exactly the one we need.

Index. Is the work indexed? Check the back of the book (or rarely, the front) to see if there is an index. Many otherwise potentially useful books are worth less than the paper they are written on because the information they contain is virtually inaccessible.

Organization. Is the book organized chronologically? Geographically? Alphabetically? By topic? Poor organization can waste much of a researcher's time. If we need information on the growth of the church in Latin America, a chronological (but not geographical) organization could waste hours of time as we have to search through data on all the other countries of the world seeking those items which refer only to Latin America. Likewise, a strictly geographical organization might not show us the progress of growth over time. In either case it might be better to find another work whose organization more exactly fit our needs.

Author's credentials. Finally, take a look at the credentials of the author. Has he or she written on this topic before?

What has his experience in the field been? Has he based his work on that of others who have been prominent in the field? If so, has he agreed or disagreed with them? Has he added to their discoveries, or merely rehashed them? How have others regarded his work? What do the critics say? If you know that the author is someone whose viewpoint is vastly different from yours, you probably won't find much support in his works for the argument you are trying to present.

While it may require a little extra effort, taking some additional time to find the appropriate book can often represent a time savings over taking the first source that comes along.

DICTIONARIES

Some major "unabridged" **dictionaries** useful to the college or university student are WEBSTER'S NEW INTERNATIONAL DICTIONARY OF THE ENGLISH LANGUAGE, WEBSTER'S THIRD NEW INTERNATIONAL DICTIONARY, or FUNK AND WAGNALL'S NEW STANDARD DICTIONARY. Actually, there are dozens of good dictionaries for student use; their major drawback is not content but lack of use.

It should be noted here that "Webster's" is a generic term coming from Noah Webster, compiler of an early dictionary, and can be used by anyone. Merriam-Webster is a reputable dictionary publisher, producer of the **Third New International Dictionary** mentioned above. If you find it confusing to distinguish one "Webster's" from another, that's just what some not-so-reputable publishers want. Just because it's a "Webster's" dictionary is no sign that it's necessarily a good one.

Major components of language dictionaries include spelling, etymologies (the history of a word), definitions, pronunciation, synonyms, syllabication, and grammatical information.

SPECIALIZED DICTIONARIES IN CRIMINAL JUSTICE

In addition to language dictionaries, there is a wide range of **specialized subject dictionaries** that the informed student will want to become acquainted with, and these may be found in the reference section.

Black, Henry Campbell. **Black's Law Dictionary**, 5th ed. St. Paul, MN: West Publishing Co., 1979.

SEARCH Group, Inc. **Dictionary of Criminal Justice Data Terminology**, 2nd ed. Washington, DC: U. S. Government Printing Office, 1981. 257 pages.

De Sola, Ralph. **Crime Dictionary**, 2nd ed. New York: Facts on File, 1988. 222 pages.

Rush, George, Eugene. **Dictionary of Criminal Justice.** Boston: Holbrook Press, 1977. 374 pages.

Williams, Vergil L. **Dictionary of American Penology: An Introductory Guide.** Westport, CT: Greenwood Press, 1979. 530 pages.

ENCYCLOPEDIAS

There is more than one kind of encyclopedia, even though many incoming students have been nurtured with the notion that either the ENCYCLOPEDIA AMERICANA or THE WORLD BOOK, or, if the student is particularly interested in specialized knowledge, the ENCYCLOPAEDIA BRITAN-NICA, constitute the full range. Wrong! Though these are very valuable sources of general information, the criminal justice student serious about library research will seek out specialized encyclopedias which will prove to be the most valuable of all. Nevertheless, general encyclopedias do have a great deal of merit.

GENERAL ENCYCLOPEDIAS

"For your research paper, you must use three different sources and you can't use an encyclopedia." Surely every student has heard this from his teacher many times over during elementary and high school. Why the bias against encyclopedias? Are they inherently evil? What's wrong with them?

Actually, nothing is basically wrong with using encyclopedias --the good ones anyway--if they are used properly. But fifth graders (and sometimes college students and graduate students) tend to rely on them too completely. Encyclopedias are often like distilled water--the essence is there, but not the flavor. Students use them heavily because they want their research pre-digested for them rather than doing it themselves from primary sources.

So, why do encyclopedias exist? Who should use them and when? How should they be used?

Encyclopedias are a ready-reference source--a handy place for quick information. They provide a broad overview of popular subjects of general interest (hence the term "general interest encyclopedia"). The articles in an encyclopedia are written by experts in the field and are aimed at those who are not.

Encyclopedias can serve the specialist by providing a summary of his or her discipline, or the novice by providing an introduction. They are a good starting point. The novice doing research on Louis XIV can get an idea of when and where he lived and who he was from the general encyclopedia. That information, at least, will tell us that we probably won't find much about him in a book on avant-garde theater in Buenos Aires, but surely will find him in books on the history of France.

If we learn from the encyclopedia that John Doe is an author and is currently living, we know to look next in reference works on contemporary authors. From the encyclopedia we learn that the haversian canals are an anatomical, not a geographical, feature and that Jeremy Bentham is a name we'll want to be on the lookout for while studying the history of criminal justice.

The encyclopedia can also be useful as a bibliographic tool. Some encyclopedias list books and articles for further reading on the topic. Check the introductory material for the encyclopedia to see if bibliographies are given and if they are with the articles or in a separate section. Rather than wonder if the library has "any books on XYZ," the prepared student will have a list of books and can go directly to the catalog to see if the library has them.

When using the encyclopedia, always approach the topic through the index, rather than by the elementary school method of grabbing the appropriate volume and looking directly for the article. Louis XIV may be listed in the "L" volume; or he may not be. But the student who looks only in the "L" volume rather than in the index will surely miss many other references to him in articles on the history of France and other topics.

Use the encyclopedia. Use it often. But use it well. And use it only as a starting point for further research.

SPECIALIZED ENCYCLOPEDIAS IN CRIMINAL JUSTICE

Bailey, William G., ed. **The Encyclopedia of Police Science.** New York: Garland Publishing, 1989. 718 pages.

Kadish, Sanford H., ed. **Encyclopedia of Crime and Justice.** New York: Free Press, 1983. 4 volumes, 1790 pages.

Kurian, George Thomas. **World Encyclopedia of Police Forces and Penal Systems.** New York: Facts on File, 1989. 582 pages.

Nash, Jay Robert. **Encyclopedia of World Crime.** Freeport, NY: Marshall Cavendish, 1989.

Scott, Harold. **The Concise Encyclopedia of Crime and Criminals.** New York: Hawthorn Books, 1961.

Sifakis, Carl. **Encyclopedia of American Crime.** New York: Facts on File, 1982. 802 pages.

GOVERNMENT DOCUMENTS

Though the government documents section of the reference collection is problematical and complex, the student of criminal justice may often need to refer to these documents. Initially, you might wish to consult one of these two sources for a general overview of the available materials, namely, Joe Morehead's INTRODUCTION TO UNITED STATES PUBLIC DOCUMENTS (Littleton, CO: Libraries Unlimited, Inc., third edition, 1983) or Laurence F. Schmeckebier and Roy B. Eastin's GOVERNMENT PUBLICATIONS AND THEIR USE (Washington, DC: The Brookings Institute, second revised edition, 1969).

An important tool used in locating United States Government documents is the MONTHLY CATALOG OF U. S. GOVERN-MENT PUBLICATIONS (U. S. Superintendent of Documents, 1895 to date) because it is the single most comprehensive listing of all unclassified publications issued by the various departments and agencies of the U. S. government. Another reference of major importance because it offers a comprehensive annotated guide to the series and periodicals produced by agencies and departments of the U. S. government is John L. Andriot's GUIDE TO U. S. GOVERNMENT PUB-LICATIONS (McLean, VA: Documents Index, 1985). For further listings, library staff will be happy to show you many of these sources and their primary method of use.

INDEXES

An indispensable category of reference works for the student of criminal justice is the indexes. Though they are too numerous for us to list all of them here, we will give a brief description of the ones most valuable to the student of criminal justice. We will include a sample entry for several of them in the **Illustrations.** Some of them index periodicals and journals and others index other reference books. There are several basic indexes every student of criminal justice should know, most of which can be found in any college library:

Bibliographic Index provides students and researchers with a useful tool to aid them in selecting information for their projects. It is a subject index to bibliographies in English and foreign languages which are found in current books and magazines. The BIBLIOGRAPHIC INDEX covers most areas in which bibliographies are compiled and offers an indication of recent scholarship and new developments in many fields. Monographs (books) are a prime source, as are the approximately 2400 periodicals which are regularly examined for bibliographies. To be listed, a bibliography must contain more than 50 citations. BIBLIOGRAPHIC INDEX is published in April and August, with a permanent bound annual cumulation in December. A sample entry is given in **Illustration 101.**

Biography Index is a guide to the location of biographical materials found in books, periodicals, and pamphlets. Access to all types of biographical writing from both primary and secondary sources is provided. These include autobiographies, bibliographies, critical studies, literature, letters, memoirs, pictoral works, and poetry. Current books of individual and collective biography in the English language are major sources, as are the more than 2400 periodicals that are given coverage for other features in the various other indexes discussed here. The obituaries in the NEW YORK TIMES are regularly included. Incidental material found in prefaces, chapters, and bibliographies of otherwise nonbiographical works are considered important sources. BIOGRAPHY INDEX consists of a main alphabetical entry by last name of the subject, with a cross reference index by profession. The index contains a checklist of composite books analyzed. Portraits and other illustrations are noted. BIOGRAPHY INDEX is published quarterly in November, February, May, and August. It is bound annually and has a permanent three-year cumulation.

Book Review Digest contains short excerpts from reviews of current books. Critical evaluations are selected from, or bibliographic references are given for, reviews appearing in 70 American, British, and Canadian periodicals. Reviews are cited for approximately 6000 books of adult and juvenile fiction and nonfiction each year. To qualify for inclusion, a book must have been either published or distributed in the United States. Each book is listed alphabetically in BOOK REVIEW DIGEST by main entry, usually the author. Title, bibliographical information, descriptive information, review excerpts, and citations follow. This main section is followed by a subject and title index. BOOK REVIEW DIGEST has quarterly cumulations and a permanent bound annual cumulation. The inclusion of excerpts from reviews often provides the needed information without making it necessary for the student to locate the actual review itself. **Illustration 102** shows an example.

Book Review Index is similar in scope and purpose to BOOK REVIEW DIGEST. The major difference is that BOOK REVIEW INDEX gives only citations for the reviews and does not include excerpts.

Criminal Justice Abstracts. (Formerly **Abstracts on Crime and Delinquency.**) Monsey, NY: Willow Tree Press, 1968-.

Criminal Justice Periodical Index. Ann Arbor, MI: University Microfilms, 1975-.

Criminology and Penology Abstracts. Amsterdam: Kugler Publishers, 1961-.

Cumulative Book Index is a current index to books published in the English language and is international in scope; 50,000 to 60,000 books are indexed each year. It is the only international index to list entries by author, title and subject in a single alphabet. The author, or main, entry includes any or all of the following pertinent bibliographic information: author's or editor's name; full title of the book; illustrator's name; translator's name; indication of illustrations or maps; binding, if other than cloth; price; International Standard Book Number (ISBN), if available; publication date; publisher; edition; series note; volume number; paging; size, if other than standard shelf size; Library of Congress card number; distributors for foreign publications available in the U. S. Each book indexed in CUMULATIVE BOOK INDEX (CBI) is cited under as many subject headings and subheadings as its contents require. Government documents, editions limited to 500 copies or fewer, inexpensive paperbound books, or materials of a local or ephemeral nature are not included.

Current Book Review Citations is an index of book reviews appearing in more than 1200 periodicals. It provides users with a guide to recent reviews of fiction and nonfiction books found in both book reviewing periodicals and subject periodicals. CURRENT BOOK REVIEW CITATIONS assists readers in keeping up with the latest critical evaluations from a wide variety of periodicals. All the major fields of intellectual and scientific pursuits are encompassed: business, education, the humanities, law, the social sciences, pure and applied sciences. Part I of CURRENT BOOK REVIEW CITATIONS is the Author Index. All book reviews are entered by the name of the author of the book reviewed. The title and the date of publication of the book are given, followed by the name of the periodical in which the review appeared with its volume number, date, and page numbers. The name of the reviewer is included if available. Part II is the Title Index. When a title is used as the main entry, the full bibliographic information is to be found in the Author Index with a "see" reference from the entry in the Title Index.

Forensic Science Abstracts: The International Medical Abstracting Services. Amsterdam: Elsevier Science Publishers, 1975-.

Index to Legal Periodicals. Bronx, NY: H. W. Wilson Co., 1908-.

Index to U. S. Government Periodicals provides a subject and author approach to 120 periodicals issued by various agencies of the Federal Government. Published quarterly, it is particularly useful for the social sciences.

PAIS (Public Affairs Information Service Bulletin) provides a selective subject listing of the latest books, pamphlets, government publications, reports of public and private agencies, and periodical articles relevant to government and public administration, international affairs, and economics. It has the advantage of relative currency since it is issued twice a month and cumulated four times a year. Retrospective searching may be accomplished through the CUMULATIVE SUBJECT INDEX TO THE PAIS ANNUAL BULLETIN (1915-1974). In addition, PAIS has been on-line since 1976. An example is provided in **Illustration 104.**

Police Science Abstracts. Amsterdam: Kugler Publishers, 1973-.

Readers' Guide To Periodical Literature. This old stand-by from high school days is still useful to the college and university student of criminal justice. Public libraries, which are often the only libraries available to the practicing professional after graduation, may not have many of the titles listed here, but most will have **Readers' Guide.** Aimed at the general public, **RG** covers a broad spectrum of journals including several titles of interest to students of criminal justice, such as **Society, Psychology Today, Time** and **USA Today**--some 200 titles altogether.

Several of those titles are of direct interest to the criminal justice community. Articles are indexed by author and subject, with entries for both located in a single alphabet. Each author and subject entry includes all the necessary bibliographic information to find the article cited: author's name, title of the article, title of the periodical, volume number, inclusive paging of the article, date of publication, and notations of illustrations, bibliographies, or other descriptive information. Book reviews are cited in a separate section. **RG** is issued twice a month with annual cumulations.

INFOTRAC II is a computerized periodicals index. One of the indexes it contains is **Magazine Index**, which is similar in scope and purpose to **Readers Guide** but published by a competitor. Running on IBM or compatible equipment, the system is simple and straightforward; the beginner can learn it in less than ten minutes. The index covers some 425 titles, including a number of journals of interest to the student of criminal justice, though its focus is on general-interest titles with an emphasis on the business world. Many of the periodicals indexed in **Readers' Guide** are also covered in Infotrac. **Infotrac** adds a decided advantage to research in that the data is stored on a compact disc (CD-ROM) and is thus accessible from more points of entry than with a manual system. The database is updated monthly and normally contains the current year plus the previous four. Some libraries also subscribe to the backfile which goes back to 1980. Citations can be sent to the attached printer, rather than hand-copied, thus reducing research time and the margin for error. It can be found in an increasing number of college and public libraries.

Several of the above indexes, and many others, are now available on-line. An increasing number of them are becoming available on CD-ROM products and are more likely than ever to be found even in smaller libraries. Ask which ones are available at your library or nearby libraries.

Some libraries subscribe to on-line services through one of the two major vendors, Dialog or BRS. Before beginning on-line research through one of the vendors, the researcher should understand something about how charges are incurred, as searching on-line can be quite expensive.

First of all is a telecommunications charge. This is the cost of the long distance phone call from the computer terminal in your library to the computer where the database is located. Most libraries will use a telecommunications network, so costs are less than for a long distance phone call, but can, nonetheless, add up.

The vendors charge for connect time, that is for the length of time the library's computer is connected to the database. These charges vary from vendor to vendor, and most greatly, from database to database. Charges range from approximately $30 per hour to more than $300 per hour. The more expensive databases tend to be those with detailed scientific information.

A third charge is per citation. That is, when the searcher requests articles on a certain topic, there is a charge for each article citation retrieved, or at least, for each citation which is printed. This charge will vary depending on how much detail is requested (for example, whether or not the citation contains an abstract of the article) or whether the citations are printed immediately on the computer screen or printer or printed off-line and mailed to the library at a later date.

Some libraries also add a surcharge per search which helps pay for some of the librarian's time; planning and executing a careful search can be very time-consuming.

Before you are scared off by the thought of paying hundreds of dollars to find a few articles, remember that the librarian is skilled at performing this type of search--some librarians more than others, so make sure you choose one who is skilled. An expert searcher can conduct the search and produce a list of articles for you in just a few seconds or minutes. (Two minutes spent in a $300 per hour database is only $10.)

It is for this reason that the librarian will usually ask you to fill out one or more forms outlining your search and the desired results as carefully as possible. He or she will usually ask you the maximum you want to spend and the number of citations you want to retrieve.

The reason for an on-line search is that it may be tailored to your needs much more carefully than a manual search. For example, you may be interested only in research that was published in the German language between 1983 and 1985. An on-line search will allow you to retrieve specifically that type of information. Assuming that you have already done a lot of research and don't need any of the articles written by John Doe, you may exclude them from your search. Or you (viz. the searcher) may program the computer to advise you each month if anything new is published in your area of interest. (This service is called SDI--Selective Dissemination of Information.)

Some of the databases of specific interest to the student of criminal justice which are now available on-line are the National Institute of Justice, LEXIS, Social SciSearch, WESTLAW, and others. Many of the other hundreds of available databases may also contain articles of interest to the criminal justice major, graduate student, or professional.

On-line searching is a terrific tool for the professional researcher. Everyone should at least be introduced to it.

Those who learn early in their career to use periodical indexes and to use them well, will find that it makes their research easier and gives it a timeliness lacking in that of many of their colleagues.

CHAPTER FOUR

PERIODICALS

Too often students are of the false impression that the library subscribes to magazines and newspapers just to keep the library user happy. That is, the magazines and various other loose items lying near and shelved close to comfortable reading desks and lounge chairs are there for the general amusement of the bored student. **NOT SO!**

From a research and scholarly point of view, there is no such thing as serious research or scholarship in the absence of the periodical literature. Furthermore, there is a profoundly important difference between the various kinds of periodical materials subscribed to by the library. To call a scholarly journal a "magazine" is a great disservice. The scholarly journal consists of heavily researched articles of a specialized nature and published for the professionals in that field.

Magazines, on the other hand, are written for the general public, the casual but interested reader, and are not research scholarship. Good magazine articles may be helpful in orienting the layman and the beginning student to the general range and nature of a topic but would never constitute the literature foundation for a serious research project. Any serious student would never refer to research scholarship in the journals as "magazine" articles. Language and terminology, as always, reflect the depth of the student's training and awareness.

The library does more than just provide copies of the latest issues of scholarly journals. It also collects the back issues and gathers them into a special collection usually in some large chamber of the library. The periodicals, therefore, are naturally divided into two categories, namely, the **Current Periodicals Section** or room and the **Bound Periodicals Section** or room. Let us discuss them in that order.

CURRENT PERIODICALS. This section of the academic library is easily identified, for here the journals, magazines, and periodical materials to which the college or university subscribes may be displayed on easy-to-get-at shelves or racks arranged so that the general reader can peruse the collection, often without having to handle each item, by reading the covers of the journals where the contents may often be listed in a convenient quick-to-use manner.

The current periodicals constitute the latest issues of a journal to which the library subscribes. The informed student researcher will make it a frequent practice to scan all of the periodicals subscribed to by the library in his own field of study and interest. By merely reading the table of contents (often printed on the cover) of the major periodicals in the field, the student can keep up with the general development of ideas and activities of his special interest.

As the current issue of a periodical is replaced by a later one, the older issue is usually placed somewhere near the latest one. Many shelves are arranged so that the older issues are kept immediately behind or under the current one. The student can locate them simply by lifting the shelf. These issues are kept together until a volume is accumulated and then sent off for binding and relocation in the Bound Periodicals Section. (A volume may constitute a year's worth of journals or perhaps only two or three months' worth. The most important criterion is keeping the bound volume of manageable size.)

BOUND PERIODICALS. There usually isn't room for the library to keep every issue of every journal to which it subscribes all together in the Current Periodicals Section, especially when one considers that there are usually several hundred subscriptions and an accumulation of many decades.

Therefore, it becomes necessary for the library to store for easy access the back issues of the major periodicals of the collection.

Virtually every academic library keeps some kind of list of its periodicals holdings. This list (which may take the form of a printed or computerized list, a card or book catalog, or a visible file) is an alphabetical listing of all the periodicals owned by the library and, just as importantly, the date the subscription commenced (and ended, if the journal is no longer received). Some collections could go back a hundred years, while others will date much more recently. This information is crucial, for it tells the student immediately whether or not a particular periodical is available in the library and at what point the subscription began (and ended).

In addition, the holdings list will tell in what form the back issues are kept. There is no use looking on the shelves if the issues are kept only in microform. Microform may be microfilm or microfiche. Some libraries may use one of the forms, while others will use the other, and some use both. It is extremely important that the student know in what form the issues are kept, for that information will determine where they are located. Though sometimes located on the shelves with the bound materials, microfilm and microfiche are usually filed in special cabinets and may be kept in a special area of the library. Film and fiche are usually kept in separate cabinets from each other.

Let us illustrate the importance of this listing. Say a student has found through the utilization of **Criminal Justice Abstracts** an excellent-sounding article on a topic of special research interest. Indexes are generic; that is, they index articles in their area of specialization without regard to the holdings of a particular library. Just because the student finds an entry in the index for an article does not mean that his library owns the journal that carries that article. Many steps and much time will be saved if the student will first check the holdings list to see if the library actually subscribes to the periodical in question and, equally important, if the subscription includes the date of the sought-after article. Without the information provided in the holdings list, the student is destined to much wasted time scurrying up and down the aisles of the Bound Periodicals Section looking for the treasure which may not even be there.

The Bound Periodicals Section may be alphabetized or classified by subject, depending upon the practice of the particular library. Some libraries may not file bound periodicals by themselves but interfile them on the shelves with the books.

In most libraries, bound periodicals stacks are open to the patron so that the student researcher is allowed to search out the needed journal issue independently. In some libraries, however, the stacks are closed and the researcher must request that the journals be brought to him.

Though we will discuss this point later, it should be emphasized here that the student must **write down legibly** the complete bibliographic information before beginning the search for needed materials. Frustration compounds confusion when the student must return again and again to the original reference in the index to get yet more information about the notation which should have been written down in its entirety at the outset.

The sad truth is that many students have only the faintest idea what the Bound Periodicals Section is or how to use it. It constitutes yet another great gray bog of mystery and superstition and, therefore, is infrequently used, particularly by the undergraduate. Too often students presume on the basis of a quick perusal of only a few current periodicals in the Current Periodicals Section, or, even worse, a casual glance through the card catalog, that the library has nothing on the subject under consideration.

The Bound Periodicals Section of the library constitutes a secret treasury which can be opened only through the use of the indexes, but once the key is discovered, namely, how to use the indexes, that great treasury willingly offers up its holdings to the earnest student.

READING A PERIODICAL. Unfortunately, students too often pass over some of the added attractions in the periodical literature. In addition to finding the especially applicable article in the scholarly journal, the observant student will find even more. First, in some scholarly journals, the articles are preceded by a substantial and very helpful **"abstract"**, a paragraph, usually in bold or italic type, which summarizes the contents of the article. The abstract will indicate immediately to the student whether this particular article is going to be of value. Often the title is not exactly descriptive of the content, but the abstract most definitely is. By reading the abstract, the student may save valuable time.

Furthermore, if a student is attempting to develop a topic by first preparing a research bibliography, there is no more effective device than finding a crucial article in the periodical literature, turning to its conclusion and finding there a well-developed bibliography already prepared by the scholar who wrote the article. Often, two or three such articles will turn up more bibliographical citations than a student can handle for a single research project. Otherwise, a student might spend hours wandering the aisles of the library "hoping" to find a bibliography on the topic at hand, never realizing that such bibliographies are there if he only knew where to look!

CHAPTER FIVE

THE RESEARCH PAPER

"...Putting It All Together..."

It has been said that the only good research paper is the written research paper. The student will discover that no matter how well the research has been executed or how profound the insight into the subject as a result of a vigorous effort in the college library, it is to no avail until the research is written up in a coherent form.

The follow-through, the **putting it all together**, is what we wish to address ourselves to in this closing chapter.

Our treatment will be brief; it will be simple but hopefully not simplistic. If the student needs more guidance than is offered here, it is available -- from the professor, from the library staff, from well written guides developed for that purpose. Substantial and detailed guides for paper-writing may be purchased in the bookstores of most universities, and the better ones are also found in most academic libraries. But for our purposes here, what follows is what we think to be a sufficient guide for the average student in the development of an above average research paper.

Essentially, two procedures are necessary in order to bring a good paper to fruition, namely, a sound search strategy for the gathering of pertinent information, and then a well developed organizational framework for the actual writing of the paper. Let us examine this process carefully.

The search strategy is a prerequisite to all research paper projects. The strategy, illustrated in the diagram provided in **Illustration** 105, consists of three primary steps.

FIRST STEP. First, in order for a student to write a research paper, he must develop a topic which derives from a subject area. Eventually, a well-thought-out topic will produce a descriptive title for the actual paper. Assuming the student has no earthly idea what to write about (not an unreasonable premise, judging from our thirty-plus years of classroom experience on both sides of the desk), finding a topic is likely to be a problem. For the student of criminal justice (or any student, for that matter), an immediate perusal of the **background sources** constitutes the first step.

The background sources are those general and specialized encyclopedias cited earlier, as well as the textbook for the course. (Students so often fail to think of the required text in the course as a primary reference, but it most certainly is!) Another, and probably more effective and time-saving method for the student of criminal justice would be to go immediately to the **Encyclopedia of Crime and Justice** that is found in the reference section of almost any college or university library. Take a volume, any volume, and thumb through it. The titles of areas of criminal justice research jump out at the reader; there are literally hundreds of possibilities, and eventually there will be a subject that even the most unanimated student will find interesting.

Good! Now, read through the article. It will probably be short and written by one of the best minds in the field. If it holds your attention, then either make a photocopy of the bibliography at the end of the article, or, if funds permit, copy the entire article, making sure to write on the first page the entire bibliographical reference, namely, the author of the essay, the title of the article, the volume, page numbers, and the date and place of publication.

Now, having first consulted the background sources and happily identified a subject area (still far removed from the final topic and title of the research paper itself, but certainly a start in the right direction), proceed to the second level of research, namely, the movement from the identification of a subject area to the development of a topic of research.

Topic Development

There are three components of the topic development area. The student will consult three very different, but related, areas of information identification. First, you will wish to consult the periodical indexes and abstracts, and as a criminal justice student, you should direct special interest and attention toward the **Criminal Justice Abstracts** (and book review indexes where applicable). In these sources you should look up articles in each of several volumes, usually beginning with the most recent volume and working backwards until a substantial amount of literature has been identified. This will vary depending on the area and the topic being pursued, of course.

You should certainly identify two dozen or more articles in the **Criminal Justice Abstracts,** checking the periodicals holdings list to make sure that the articles that are included in the developing bibliography for the research paper are actually available in the college or university library. (If they are not, and if there is sufficient time, the student can always call for these articles through the Interlibrary Loan Department). The subjects chosen while perusing the **Encyclopedia of Crime and Justice** should be identified by one, two, or three words, called "key word indicators." These words should be looked up in **Criminal Justice Abstracts,** for example, such key words as police, courts, corrections, and organized crime.

SECOND STEP. The next step in the search strategy is to consult the **BIBLIOGRAPHIC INDEX** and look up the key word indicators to see if there is already a well developed and reasonably recent bibliography on the subject area that you are interested in pursuing. If so, much of your work has already been done, for the development of an effective bibliography constitutes a major component in any research effort.

Finally, after gathering two dozen articles from the **Criminal Justice Abstracts** (making sure to get complete bibliographic information and not using any abbreviations, but writing out every word completely), go to the card catalog and look up the key words on the subject cards for a listing of books and related materials held in the library stacks.

Before proceeding to the third step in this search strategy model, we feel compelled to say more at this point about the notes being taken. You, obviously, are not yet taking notes on the research topic since it is not yet well developed. However, you should be armed with a stack of 3 x 5 cards upon which each bibliographic reference is written -- only one reference per card! The complete bibliographic notation should include author, article title, periodical title, volume, issue number, date, and pages, as well as the source of the reference, in this instance the **Criminal Justice Abstracts** indicating which volume and page number. If you don't take down this information in its entirety, more than likely much time will be taken up in wasted steps retracing search procedures and countless hours spent redoing what should have been done in the first place.

It is a good idea to have a standard form on which to record the needed information. **Illustration 106** provides a suggested format for such a card. You may wish to duplicate a number of these cards ahead of time and then when a reference is found, just fill in the information, remembering to avoid abbreviations. (This point about not abbreviating is being belabored here for a purpose. For example, if you record from the **Criminal Justice Abstracts** a reference to a splendid article in the **JQ** periodical and record the reference as such, by the time you get to the bound periodicals area, you may have forgotten the exact and complete title of that specific reference. Then what? Probably a retracing of the reference by means of returning to the **Criminal Justice Abstracts** and checking the reference index to find out that **JQ** is **Justice Quarterly.** If the full title had been recorded once and first, no retracing would need occur -- resulting in much time saved!)

Again, the student should be reminded that in the front of all reference indexes, in this instance the **Criminal Justice Abstracts** there is a directory to the abbreviations used in the body of the index which you may refer to if in doubt about the correct and full title of certain periodicals. Remember that these cards will later serve as the master bibliographic file when you are writing the actual paper and, if you make them complete from the outset, they will constitute a major help in subsequent writing.

THIRD STEP. Step three in the search strategy model is actually using the sources of information, namely the periodicals and the books identified in the preceeding step. The books can be taken out of the library (unless they are categorized as rare books or reference works). The periodical literature usually may not be. However, most college and university libraries have copying facilities at minimal cost. Students are wise to copy the major articles to be used in their research, thus allowing them to move about with their research portfolio. Otherwise, the note-taking step must occur within the confines of the library, probably in the bound periodicals area.

The search has ended. The materials have been identified. This process, once rehearsed, can be executed in an hour or so. We know for a fact (as judged from experience) that a student who has been trained in this system of library usage skills can enter the library without any notion of a topic and in less than an hour develop quite a respectable working bibliography.

FROM CHAOS TO ORDER. At this juncture, you must begin to concentrate seriously upon the organizational model of the research. Our experience leads us to propose this model. At this point you have moved from no subject area to the discovery, thanks to the **Encyclopedia of Crime and Justice,** of a viable and interesting subject area.

Furthermore, you have developed the subject area, owing to the three-fold utilization of the search strategy model with the **Criminal Justice Abstracts,** the **BIBLIOGRAPHIC INDEX** and the card catalog, into an identifiable topic, and have a working bibliography to prove it. Now, you must become acquainted with the materials appropriate to the topic which have been identified, gleaned, and collected. We propose the following process:

KNOWING AND OWNING THE MATERIALS

A.   QUICK PERUSAL. Now you should quickly peruse all materials (two dozen articles or so, plus a particularly appropriate book or two on the topic -- articles, not books, you will find, constitute the substance of library research in criminal justice). If you have photocopies of the articles, they should be discreetly underlined and marked at particularly important points. The idea here is a general acquaintance with the materials.

B.   OUTLINE DEVELOPMENT. You should now develop an outline. Most research papers at this level will have three to five major components with three or four sub-headings under each of those. Without an outline, the paper can hardly have a sense of developed logic and reasoned organization to it. Writing the outline after the paper has already been written is like drawing up architectural plans for a house already constructed. The purpose of the outline is to help you develop the topic.

C.   READ CAREFULLY. Following the development of the outline (based on your knowledge of the materials gained in A. above) with a second and more careful reading of the collected materials is a must. Here, you should be armed with a good supply of 3 x 5 cards. At each opportunity, when you identify something of noteworthy importance to the topic at hand, it should be written down. One quotation or one notation per card. Never two or more! This is the wisest rule to follow because, later, the student who has foolishly recorded two or three important quotations on a single card may find that one quotation will go in one stack for one point and another quotation (from the same card) will need to go into another stack for a different point. One note per card is imperative.

Furthermore, on each card, you must indicate at the top left-hand corner, the author, short-word title of the article and page number. If this information is not written down on each card as the note is being taken, then the chances of the cards getting mixed up are overwhelming. When the cards are mixed inadvertently, no matter how excellent the notations, the student has no idea of the source of the note or the quotation, thus rendering this particular card invalid.

D. REVISE AND EXPAND. After you have gleaned all the notes and quotations from the materials gathered for the project, then the outline developed in B. above must be revised and expanded to incorporate every aspect of the research materials which you wish to include. This usually means 1) a minor rewording and/or reworking of the major headings and sub-headings, and 2) the further development of the sub-headings which will provide a means of incorporating most of the notes and quotations taken in C. above.

E. CARDS AND OUTLINE. This next to the last step is crucial. You should take the outline in its final developed form placing the stack of note cards beside the outline. Now, taking the cards as a deck of playing cards, label each card in the upper right-hand corner (remember the author/short title/page number is in the upper left-hand corner) with a Roman numeral corresponding to the major headings of the outline, that is, I, II, III, IV, V, etc. You need to go through the entire stack of cards, labeling them with a major heading number and placing each in its appropriate stack.

Now you will have three or four or five large separate stacks of research cards. That task being accomplished, take stack I (the first major division within the outline) and proceeding through just this stack alone, mark each card with a sub-heading: A., B., C., D., E., F., etc., which corresponds to the sub-headings in the outline under Roman numeral I.

After completing the labeling of the first stack with the sub-heading letters, you should proceed to the second and subsequent stacks until all major heading stacks have been divided into the sub-heading stacks.

Finally, assuming that you have wisely developed sub-subheadings (this third level indicates excellence in organization with the sub-headings often corresponding to individual paragraphs within the finished paper) the cards in the subheadings should be divided into sub-sub-heading stacks. That being done, you now have all cards categorized into just their appropriate place within the paper. For example, if your paper has three major components, I, II, and III, and each of these has three sub-headings, A., B., and C., and each of these has three sub-sub-headings, 1., 2., and 3., you will have divided the research cards first into three stacks corresponding to I., II., and III., and then into nine stacks corresponding to I.A., I.B., I.C., II.A., II.B., II.C., III.A., III.B., and III.C. Finally, you will sub-divide these nine stacks into three stacks each corresponding to I.A.1., I.A.2., I.A.3., I.B.1., I.B.2., I.B.3., etc. The smaller the stack, the smaller the category of treatment, thereby making the paper develop in its writing in small careful steps versus wild sporadic steps undisciplined by an outline and organized notecards! (The reason for placing only one bit of information on a single card and identifying that card with author/title/page now becomes apparent.)

F. NUMBER THE CARDS. Now, before an accident occurs and all the cards fall to the floor or maybe get dropped on campus, you should turn the cards over and number them consecutively from the first to the very last card. Since they are in exactly the proper order for the writing, this precautionary measure is strictly protective. Now, if they are dropped on the floor or while walking across campus, they can easily and quickly be put back into their proper sequencing.

G. WRITE THE PAPER. This, of course, is the whole purpose of the exercise. You need to line up the cards consecutively, beginning with number one, and put the information from each card, whether note or quotation, into a coherent style of writing, quoting where needed and paraphrasing otherwise. In no time at all, the paper is completed and a successful research project brought to completion.

BIBLIOGRAPHY

BIBLIOGRAPHIES

Davis, Bruce L. **Criminological Bibliographies: Uniform Citations to Bibliographies, Indexes, and Review Articles of the Literature of Crime Study in the United States.** Westport, CT: Greenwood Press, 1978. 182 pages.

Klein, Carol and David M. Horton. **Bibliographies in Criminal Justice: A Selected Bibliography.** Washington, DC: National Institute of Justice, 1980.

DICTIONARIES

Black, Henry Campbell. **Black's law Dictionary**, 5th ed. St. Paul, MN: West Publishing Co., 1979.

SEARCH Group, Inc. **Dictionary of Criminal Justice Data Terminology**, 2nd ed. Washington, DC: U. S. Government Printing Office, 1981. 257 pages.

De Sola, Ralph. **Crime Dictionary**, 2nd ed. New York: Facts on File, 1988. 222 pages.

Rush, George, Eugene. **Dictionary of Criminal Justice.** Boston: Holbrook Press, 1977. 374 pages.

Williams, Vergil L. **Dictionary of American Penology: An Introductory Guide.** Westport, CT: Greenwood Press, 1979. 530 pages.

ENCYCLOPEDIAS

Bailey, William G., ed. **The Encyclopedia of Police Science.** New York: Garland Publishing, 1989. 718 pages.

Kadish, Sanford H., ed. **Encyclopedia of Crime and Justice.** New York: Free Press, 1983. 4 volumes, 1790 pages.

Kurian, George Thomas. **World Encyclopedia of Police Forces and Penal Systems.** New York: Facts on File, 1989. 532 pages.

Nash, Jay Robert. **Encyclopedia of World Crime.** Freeport, NY: Marshall Cavendish, 1989.

Scott, Harold. **The Concise Encyclopedia of Crime and Criminals.** New York: Hawthorn Books, 1961.

Sifakis, Carl. **The Encyclopedia of American Crime.** New York: Facts on File, 1982. 802 pages.

HANDBOOKS AND YEARBOOKS

Johnson, Elmer, ed. **International Handbook of Contemporary Developments in Criminology.** Westport, CT: Greenwood Press, 1983. 2 volumes.

Morris, Norval and Michael Tonry, eds. **Crime and Justice: An Annual Review of Research.** Chicago: University of Chicago Press, 1979-.

Sage Criminal Justice System Annuals. Beverly Hills: Sage Publications, 1972-.

Wright, Martin. **Use of Criminological Literature.** Hamden, CT: Archon Books, 1974. 242 pages.

OTHER REFERENCES

Andriot, John L. **Guide to U. S. Government Publications.** McLean, VA: Documents Index, 1985.

Gates, Jean Key. **Guide to the Use of Libraries and Information Sources,** 6th edition. New York: McGraw-Hill, 1988.

Morehead, Joe. **Introduction to United States Public Documents.** Littleton, CO: Libraries Unlimited, Inc., 1983, third edition, 309 pp.

Schmeckebier, Laurence F. and Roy B. Eastin. **Government Publications and Their Use.** Second revised edition, Washington, DC: The Brookings Institute, 1969. 502 pp.

INDEXES

Bibliographic Index

Biography Index

Book Review Digest

Book Review Index

Criminal Justice Abstracts. (Formerly **Abstracts on Crime and Delinquency.**) Monsey, NY: Willow Tree Press, 1963-.

Criminal Justice Periodical Index. Ann Arbor, MI: University Microfilms, 1975-.

Criminology and Penology Abstracts. Amsterdam: Kugler Publishers, 1961-.

Cumulative Book Index

Current Book Review Citations

Foreign Language Index

Forensic Science Abstracts: The International Medical Abstracting Services. Amsterdam: Elsevier Science Publishers, 1975-.

Index to Legal Periodicals. Bronx, NY: H. W. Wilson Co., 1908-.

Index to U. S. Government Periodicals

PAIS (Public Affairs Information Service Bulletin)

Police Science Abstracts. Amsterdam: Kugler Publishers, 1973-.

Readers Guide to Periodical Literature. NY: Wilson, 1900-.

INFOTRAC II

ON-LINE INDEXES

Document Retrieval Index of the National Criminal Justice Reference Service. Rockville, MD: NCJRS, 1972-.

Law Enforcement and Criminal Justice Information Database. Eagan, MN: International Research and Evaluation, 1954-.

Legal Resource Index. American Association of Law Libraries, 1980-.

LEXIS. Dayton, OH: Mead Data Central, Inc. 1985-.

NCJRS Electronic Bulletin Board. Rockville, MD: National Criminal Justice Reference Service.

Social Sciences Index. Bronx, NY: H. W. Wilson Company, 1984-. Host: WilsonLine.

Social SciSearch. Philadelphia: Institute for Scientific Information, 1972-. Hosts: BRS, Data-Star, DIALOG, DIMDI, TECH DATA.

Sociological Abstracts. San Diego: Sociological Abstracts, Inc. 1963-. Hosts: BRS, Data-Star, DIALOG, TECH DATA.

The United Nations Criminal Justice Information Network. Albany, NY: United Nations, 1989-.

WESTLAW. St. Paul, MN: West Publishing Company, 1980-.

STATISTICS SOURCES

Drugs and Crime Data Center Clearinghouse. **Federal Drug Data for National Policy.** Rockville, MD: D&CDC, 1990.

CJAIN: The Criminal Justice Archive and Information Network. Ann Arbor, MI: CJAIN.

FBI. **Uniform Crime Reports: Crime in the United States.** Washington, DC: U. S. Government Printing Office, 1930-.

National Institute of Justice. **Report to the Nation on Crime and Justice.** 2nd ed. Washington, DC: U. S. Government Printing Office, 1988.

National Institute of Justice. **Sourcebook of Criminal Justice Statistics.** Washington, DC: U. S. Government Printing Office, 1973-.

MAJOR CRIMINAL JUSTICE PERIODICALS

American Journal of Criminal Justice

Crime and Delinquency

Crime and Social Justice: Issues in Criminology

Crime Control Digest

Criminal Justice and Behavior

Criminal Justice Ethics

Criminal Justice Newsletter

Criminal Justice Policy Review

Criminal Justice Review

Criminology: An Interdisciplinary Journal

Journal of Contemporary Criminal Justice

Journal of Crime and Justice

Journal of Criminal Law and Criminology

Journal of Research in Crime and Delinquency

Justice Professional

Justice Quarterly

ABOUT THE AUTHORS

Dennis C. Tucker, series editor of the Library Research Skills Series, holds a B.S. in education from Southeast Missouri State University, an M.A.T. in English from Southeast Missouri, and an M.L.S. from the University of Missouri. He has served as reference librarian at the University of Notre Dame, as Director of Library Services at Bethel College in Mishawaka, Indiana, and is currently Library Microcomputer Specialist for The Indiana Cooperative Library Services Authority (INCOLSA).

Frank Schmalleger, Ph.D. is chair of the Department of Sociology, Social Work, and Criminal Justice at Pembroke State University in North Carolina. Author of many books, including the introductory textbook **Criminal Justice Today** (Prentice Hall, 1991), he also serves as editor of the Prentice Hall series "Criminal Justice in the Twenty-First Century." As co-editor of **The Social Basis of Criminal Justice** (University Press of America, 1981), and founding editor of the journal **The Justice Professional**, Schmalleger has worked to raise ethical concerns within the justice field.

APPENDICES

Illustration

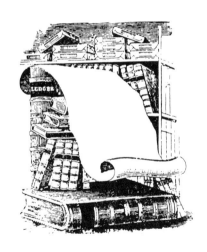

ILLUSTRATION 101

BIBLIOGRAPHIC INDEX

istration of

revention

eterrence
on. National Crime Prevention

: and its victims; what we can
W. Colson. InterVarsity Press

participation

ograms
iblic and crime prevention; a
terature. (Public administration
3) Vance Bibls. 1989 6p
iany (West)
Wallraff-Unzicker, Franziska.
ıls gesamtgesellschaftliche Auf-
lundeskriminalamtes Wiesbaden
987: Literaturzusammenstellung;
Friedhelm Berckhauer. (COD-
skriminalamt 1987 257p
at Britain
ne prevention measures. (Home
86) H.M.S.O. 1985 p69-75
ee Crime and the press
Crime scene searches

:rs. Techniques of crime scene
ord by Sherman Block. 4th ed

statistics
d mystery stories

banner of battle; the story of
rtin's Press 1987 p273-8
crimes and offenses
imes

law)
ged—Crimes against
nen—Crimes against
Criminal law
crimes

Statistics
See Criminal statistics
Criminal insane *See* **Insane, Criminal and dangerous**
Criminal investigation
See also
Burglary investigation
Child abuse—Investigation
Crime scene searches
Legal documents—Identification
Lie detectors and detection
Medical jurisprudence
Writing—Identification
Fisher, Barry A. J., and others. Techniques of crime scene investigation; with a foreword by Sherman Block. 4th ed Elsevier 1987 p503-14
Criminal justice, Administration of
See also
Corrections
Crime and criminals
Criminal investigation
Criminal law
Criminal procedure
Discrimination in criminal justice administration
Home detention
Imprisonment
Juvenile justice, Administration of
Law enforcement
Police
Prisons
Probation
Prosecution
Punishment
Rehabilitation of criminals
Sex discrimination in criminal justice administration
Douglas, R. Tolerated contests? plea and sentence in the Victorian magistrates' courts. *J Crim Justice* 16 no4:289-90 '88
Elias, Robert. The politics of victimization; victims, victimology, and human rights. Oxford Univ. Press 1986 p246-372 annot
Goehlert, Robert. Basic research resources in criminal justice. (Public administration series, bibliography P-2023) Vance Bibls. 1986 12p
Jünger, M. Racial discrimination in criminal justice in the Netherlands. *Sociol Soc Res* 72:214-16 Jl '88
Kempf, K. L. Delinquency: do the dropouts drop back in? *Youth Soc* 20:286-9 Mr '89
Wilbanks, William. The myth of a racist criminal justice system. Brooks/Cole 1987 p172-200
Bibliography
The Encyclopedia of police science; editor, William G. Bailey; editorial board members, Victor G. Strecher [et al.]. Garland 1988 p701-4
Citizen participation
Informal justice?; edited by Roger Matthews. Sage Publs. 1988 p199-211
Statistics
See Criminal statistics
Alaska
History
Stone, Thomas. Miners' justice; migration, law, and order on the Alaska-Yukon frontier, 1873-1902. (American university studies, Series XI, Anthropology/Sociology, v34) Lang, P. 1988 p284-302

ILLUSTRATION 102

BOOK REVIEW DIGEST

ZIMRING, FRANKLIN E.—*Continued*
"Using an advocacy scholarship perspective, Zimring and Hawkins examine—in a powerful, responsive, and lucid fashion—the issues and concerns surrounding the death penalty and its imposition in the US and Western industrialized nations. An insightful analysis unfolds the penalty's symbolic aspects, and accounts for general populist support, dynamics related to execution rates, eight Amendment and Supreme Court decisions (with valuable examinations of Furman versus Georgia, 1972, and Gregg versus Georgia, 1976), and connections between murder, sentencing, and penal policy. . . . This study offers original, analytical, and logical challenges to the symbolic and actual use of the death penalty and shows why American society must eliminate it as punishment for civil crimes. . . . Recommended for academic libraries, community college level up."
Choice 25:228 S '87. J.H. Larson (180w)

"[This book] makes for extremely lively reading about an otherwise 'tired subject.' . . . Further reflection about the past (and future) battles that may accelerate, shape, or retard the judicial, historical, and political events that are described as contributing to the abolitionist movement would have been beneficial. . . . The dreams and prognostications about the death penalty that may be found in this book are speculative but engaging; had they ranged to do more active battle they could have been compelling."
Contemp Sociol 17:67 Ja '88. James R. Acker (700w)

"No one seriously interested in the death penalty controversy can afford to overlook this important book."
Libr J 112:81 Ja '87. Edward C. Dreyer (120w)

Readings 3:13 S '88. Richard R. Korn (1650w)

Society 26:[84] N/D '88. Nathaniel J. Pallone (2100w)

ZIMRING, FRANKLIN E. The citizen's guide to gun control; [by] Franklin E. Zimring [and] Gordon Hawkins. 201p il $17.95 1987 Macmillan
    363.33 1. Firearms—Law and legislation 2. Crime
    ISBN 0-02-934830-7   LC 87-5503

Beginning with "chapters on the relationships between firearms and violence in the US, the authors move to a discussion of patterns of gun ownership and use. They proceed with an examination of gun control legislation at the federal, state, and local levels, and the impact of the Second Amendment on such legislation, and they conclude with a look to the future of gun control in the US." (Choice) Bibliography. Index.

"This small volume plus . H. Rossi's Under the Gun [I Considered Dangerous [BRD best comprehensive reviews Taken together, the three v balanced introduction to the
Libr J 112:89 Jl '87. J

"This topic of perennial ir thoroughly, simply, and open fully address all the arguments studies and statistics in a r multitude of charts and graph forces readers to carefully c light of statistical data. Ther to the problem and students on which to base opinions.'
SLJ 34:97 F '88. Dorca

ZINDEL, PAUL. The amaz of Eugene Dingman. 186p Harper & Row
    ISBN 0-06-026862-X; 0-(
    LC 82-47712
"A Charlotte Zolotow b

"At fifteen, Eugene is sent at an Adirondack hotel, anc . . Grades seven to ten." (

"While fiction in diary forn adults, it's hard to get right self-dramatization and irreleva slips in both directions, but, o . . . The entries are a mix of gc headlines, tales of misadventu to a beautiful but heartless . . the ache to talk to his fat Eugene was nine. The humo the pathos tugs too hard, bu tormentors (including himself fying."
Bull Cent Child Books 4 (100w)

"[Eugene] sounds and act Adolescent trauma is his lif in diary format, this is aut rambling. Readers will have out the story, and when Euge 'born' at the end, they will
SLJ 34:142 O '87. John

ILLUSTRATION 103

CRIMINAL JUSTICE ABSTRACTS

584   Criminal Justice Abstracts, December 1989

Police

1278-21
Fooner, Michael. *Interpol: issues in world crime and international criminal justice.* New York and London: Plenum, 1989. 244p. [R 48760]

A study analyzes the history and present policies of the International Criminal Police Organization (Interpol). Topics include Interpol's identity, governance, operations and management.

Interpol was formed in 1923 by police chiefs from 20 countries. In the 1920s and 1930s, Interpol developed its multinational police cooperation system at a time when counterfeiting was a major international crime problem. Although initially cautious about using its resources against international terrorism because of its political overtones, in the past decade Interpol has adopted more aggressive policies against terrorism and money laundering. What is distinctive is Interpol's approach to crime problems through orderly application of rules that are based on a consensus derived from universal principles of human rights. For example, its "terrorism defining procedure" excludes political insurgents whose actions take place against opponents (rather than uninvolved citizens) in their own nations.

1279-21
Dunford, Franklyn W.; Huizinga, David; Elliott, Delbert S. "The Omaha domestic violence police experiment." Unpublished, 1989. 67p. App. [R 48973] Prepared for the U.S. National Institute of Justice.

The Omaha Domestic Violence Police Experiment was designed, along with 5 other projects funded by the U.S. National Institute of Justice, to replicate the Minneapolis Domestic Violence Experiment. The latter concluded that arrest was the most effective of the methods used by police to reduce domestic violence. Following the design used in Minneapolis, in Omaha misdemeanor domestic violence assault cases were randomly assigned to arrest (N=109), separation (N=106) and mediation (N=115) dispositions where both suspects and victim were present when police arrived. If suspects were absent when police arrived, cases were randomly assigned to a "warrant" (N=111) or "no

ILLUSTRATION 104

PUBLIC AFFAIRS INFORMATION SERVICE
BULLETIN

Interstate cooperation

Abell, Richard B. Effective systems for regional intelligence sharing. *Police Chief 55:58-9 N '88*
Seven multistate projects that facilitate criminal information exchange; US.

CRIMINAL JURISDICTION

Bishop, Donna M. and others. Prosecutorial waiver: case study of a questionable reform. bibl tables *Crime and Delinquency 35:179-201 Ap '89*
Waiver which allows prosecutors to choose whether to initiate proceedings in juvenile or criminal court; examines the practice in Florida.

CRIMINAL JUSTICE

See also
Directories - Criminal justice.
Juvenile justice.
Sentences (law)

† Baumann, Fred E. and Kenneth M. Jensen, ed. Crime and punishment: issues in criminal justice. '89 ix+132p table indexes (LC 88-25854) (ISBN 0-8139-1191-5) pa $10.95—*Univ Pr Va*
Based on a conference sponsored by the Public Affairs Conference Center, Kenyon College, 1983. Models of punishment based on retribution and rehabilitation; US.

Bidinotto, Robert James. Crime and consequences. il *Freeman 39:252-62 Jl, 294-304 Ag, 340-51 S '89*
Argues that the US criminal justice system makes excuses for criminals instead of holding them responsible for their actions.

Downes, David. Contrasts in tolerance: post-war penal policy in the Netherlands and England and Wales. '88 x+226p bibl tables chart index (Oxford socio-legal studies) (LC 88-5264) (ISBN 0-19-825608-6) $55 —*Oxford Univ Pr*

Galaway, Burt. Restitution as innovation or unfilled promise? bibl tables *Federal Probation 52:3-14 S '88*
Review of practices since the establishment of the Minnesota Restitution Center in 1972; based on conference paper.

Gest, Ted and others. Victims of crime: the nation's crime siege has continued through the 1980s despite predictions it would ease. il table *U S News 107:16-19 Jl 31 '89*
Inability of the justice system to punish perpetrators; US.

Izvestia round table: Crime is a cause of alarm in·society. *Current Dig Soviet Pr 41:23-5+ Je 21 '89*
Condensed and translated from Izvestia, May 23, 1989.
Factors in USSR crime increase; discussion by law enforcement officials and legal scholars.

Jackson, Michael. Locking up natives in Canada. *Univ*

New York (state). Criminal Justic of Policy Analysis, Research, a Crime and justice annual report tables charts map (13th an. rep *Tower, Stuyvesant Plaza, Alban*

† Plas, Adèle G. van der. Revolutio the Cuban experiment, 1959-19 chart (Latin Am. studies 39) (I! 37.50 guilders ($18.75)—*Foris*
Published by the Center for I Research and Documentation.
Translated from the Dutch b) Emergence and integration in base tribunals.

Rosenbaum, Jill Leslie, ed. Specia crime. bibls tables *Crime and D '89*
Female offending and the crir response to women, with empha of the role of the family; US, ch

† Scott, Joseph E. and Travis Hirsch issues in crime and justice. '88 ' (Studies in crime, law and justic 87-27333) (ISBN 0-8039-2912-9 0-8039-2913-7) pa—*Sage Pubns*
Issues in policing, the courts, including alternatives to prison; US.

Stekette, Gail and Anne H. Austir justice system: utilization and in *63:285-303 Je '89*
Examines the research literatu decisions to report the crime an assailants; US.

Wheeler, Gerald R. and Rodney V time analysis of criminal sanctio offenders: a case for alternatives tables charts *Evaluation R 12:51*
The effects of fine, probation, recidivism; based on a three yea involving offenders charged in J: Texas.

† Wright, Martin and Burt Galaway, criminal justice: victims, offende viii+280p bibls charts index (L(0-8039-8063-9) $47.50; (ISBN 0 $18.95—*Sage Pubns*
Assesses the experience of me in practice, in North America, V Japan.

Costs

Strasser, Fred. Making the punishn the prison budget: it's the secon in sentencing policy that has swe

ILLUSTRATION 105

SEARCH STRATEGY MODEL

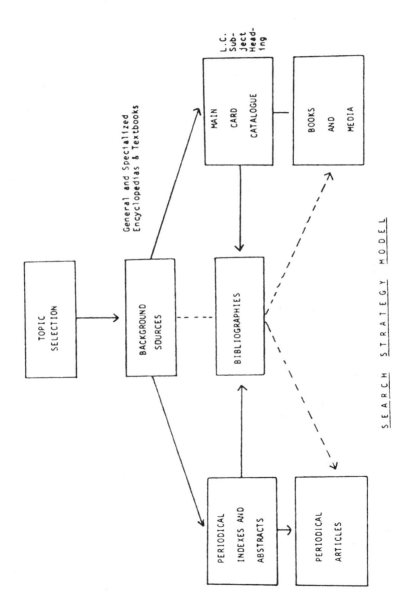

ILLUSTRATION 106

BIBLIOGRAPHIC NOTE CARD

Author (s) _____

Title of article _____

Journal title _____

Vol. _____ No. _____ Month _____ Year _____ Pages _____

Place of publication, publisher, date, edition (books only)
_____

Library where info. is located _____ Call No. _____

Source of bibliographic info. _____

How item relates to research problem _____

Use reverse side for additional comment. (if used, check here) ☐

DATE DUE
